THE ART AND SCIENCE OF BEING STILL

Using the Power of Silence for Mental, Emotional and Spiritual Health and Healing.

DOUGLAS D ZACCANELLI

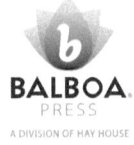

BALBOA.
PRESS
A DIVISION OF HAY HOUSE

Balboa Press books may be ordered through booksellers or by contacting:

Balboa Press
A Division of Hay House
1663 Liberty Drive
Bloomington, IN 47403
www.balboapress.com
1 (877) 407-4847

Print information available on the last page.

ISBN: 978-1-5043-9292-1 (sc)
ISBN: 978-1-5043-9293-8 (e)

Balboa Press rev. date: 01/26/2018

The foundation and lowest common denominator of our human existence is our thoughts, they alone have almost absolute power and dominion over our lives.

For Hans Olsen, my teacher.
and John Methusula, his teacher
and John's teacher who dwelt in a cave in the Himalayas.
Without them this work would not exist!

Most of us are completely unaware of the almost absolute power and influence that our thoughts have in our lives.

Foreword

The other day, my wife and I were walking to our car after grocery shopping, There was a guy just sitting in his car next to ours and as we approached he got out of his car and came towards us. I had no idea what he could have wanted but it was obvious he was waiting there for us or me actually. He said, "you probably don't remember me but I was in your Being Still class at the VA a couple months ago. I just wanted to thank you again for what you taught me". He went on to explain how much better he felt and how much better his life is now and how much he had to look forward to. He thanked me again and left. My wife commented that he looked very happy and healthy. I would have to say he looked like he finally had it back together.

For many years I have been teaching a class I call "Stop the Thoughts" at the VA Hospital in Battle Creek, Michigan. The class has also been called Being Still. I changed the name a while back because of a universal thought that everyone has when dealing with depression. That universal thought that many of us have goes something like, "if I could just stop these thoughts, everything would be fine". That thought is true and reason and intelligence tells us that it is. The roots and cause of depression is in our conscious thoughts and not in the subconscious or unconscious as many teach and believe. I will dispell that theory in this book. Another reason that I changed the name is because some thought the class to be just another method of meditation, which it is not. The difference between the Being Still exercise and meditation makes all of the difference in healing.

It only takes me a few minutes to teach someone how to be still. During the other forty or so minutes I explain why and how the Being Still mental exercise is so effective in stopping those obtrusive thoughts. I teach some things that are very obvious, yet they are either missed, ignored or outright denied in the conventional paths of treatment. I watch heads nod as I ask them how they can expect those depressive thoughts to go away if they keep thinking and talking about them all of the time. I tell them why their depressive thoughts are sometimes worse after therapy. I then explain why they will never think, talk, therapy, medicate or meditate their way out of depression. Most of what I teach is diametrically opposite to the way psychology and science thinks and teaches. After explaining what is really going on in their head, it becomes easy to explain why Being Still will be so effective in helping them free themselves from their misery.

This little book explains in a comprehensive and definitive way all that most people with depression, PTSD and many of the other maladies associated with depression needs to know and understand. Depression and all of the maladies that stem from it including PTSD and substance abuse are some of the worst wounds that we can bare.

It is important to understand that all of those conditions are rooted in depression and depression is rooted in our thoughts, our conscious, moment to moment, everyday thoughts!

I can't believe it was that simple.

A Vietnam Veteran

(Two weeks after he was taught how to be still and
after more than 40 years of suffering from PTSD)

Contents

The Science of Mind and Thought

The Effects of your Attention

Here is a practical example;

Thoughts become intrusive in the same way a fantasy that you have thought a lot about does.

Remember how the fantasy just wouldn't go away when you decide to stop thinking it.

Remember how you had to avoid thinking about the fantasy for it to go away?

<u>This book explains why that fantasy wouldn't go away.</u>
<u>It also explains how intrusive thoughts act</u>
<u>in the same way as fantasy thoughts.</u>

LET US REASON
TOGETHER FOR
A MOMENT

Let's set aside our belief that the conventional and time honored ways of working it out through thinking and talking about it can actually work.

Have you ever wondered what would have happened to you if you had spent as much time thinking and talking about some goals you had set for yourself, instead of spending all of that time with your depressive thoughts?

Instead of being more depressed wouldn't you be happy, rich, beautiful, smart, strong and have a romantic relationship with the most beautiful person imaginable!

Seriously, why should we expect that thinking and talking about either of the two, our goals or our depressive thoughts, would have any other effect then intensifying and manifesting them?

You really are what you think and you and the life you are living is becoming what you think about most, and it follows that you certainly are creating your own heaven or hell, happiness or misery in and through the thoughts that you spend your day thinking.

Depression and many of the conditions associated with it, or caused by it, are not so much psychological issues as they are thought issues.

How many times have you said to yourself?

"If I could just stop these thoughts, everything would be fine."

You should instinctively know in your heart and mind that that thought is true and reason tells you that it is true.

The bases or root of depression and
the maladies associated with it is
in your conscious thoughts.

For as he thinketh in his heart, so is he:

Proverbs 23:7 King James Bible

How we are unconsciously creating the life we are living.

Many of us know that to get where we want to go in life it is vastly important to set goals and work toward them. We need to think often about our goals, write them down, post them and visit them often. Some of us even visualize them; we spend time holding the picture of what we want in our mind. The more effective we are at doing these things the quicker they become manifested in our lives. The thoughts that we think is the way that we all, every single one of us, have created the life that we have.

Whether we are aware of it or not, we and the life we are living and who and what we will become begins within our mind. Every one of our thoughts contributes to who and what we are and who and what we are becoming. Our thoughts become manifested in our lives because that is how we and the life we experience are created. The life we experience is created through our thoughts and through our actions as they are in harmony with our thoughts. Even those who know this are not fully aware of how much influence and power each and every thought has in their lives. Life is all, every bit of it, about and because of the conscious thoughts that we think as much as the things said and the actions we perform. Whether you know it or not does not matter, the reality of life is that you and your thoughts are continuously self-involved in self-creating the life that you are living. If you doubt this, spend some time thinking about it.

This dynamic of the creation of your life from the thoughts you have holds true in every situation, any thoughts you have and especially those thoughts held in mind or continuously visited will manifest themselves in your life. It is only reasonable to realize that in the same way that your goals become manifest because of your constant thinking, talking and visualizing them, the same effect will happen of the thoughts that bring you into depression.

As you allow yourself to continuously think destructive and self-defeating thoughts they will manifest themselves in your life in the same way that goals do. Your life is made out of your thoughts, the structure or material that those thoughts are made of is the same in both instances, and the only difference between thoughts is the content of the thought. While the thoughts containing the goals you desire and think about bring about a degree of wanted results, the negative and self-defeating thoughts you constantly think will bring about their content as well. Depressive thoughts and talking about it will bring depression and all of the destructive effects that come with it, including the eventual development of uncontrollable and intrusive thoughts.

Whether battling depression or seeking the realization of lofty goals, as in any pursuit we aim our thoughts and mind at, our condition is the realization of what we have spent so much of our time thinking about. Our lives are driven primarily by our thoughts, followed by words and actions. As a person with depression spends so much time dwelling on the thoughts that accompany that condition and then is encouraged to talk about it and explore the so called triggers and the other possible subconscious or unconscious causes of it, the condition will only worsen.

Thinking and talking about it, including therapy, has and will only make it worse.

Therapy is a valuable tool in helping people with certain psychological conditions, such as personality disorders or behavior problems and it is effective in helping people to understand themselves better, mending or improving relationships and helping families to interact. But therapy, while may be helpful in the beginning, quickly becomes counterproductive in trying to alleviate the problems with depression.

Taking the former points made here under consideration, it should become increasingly obvious that it is impossible to think or talk your way out of depression. Thinking about it constantly, talking about it with others and therapy not only feeds the thoughts that cause depression but can also have an agitating effect on the mind.

Agitation in the mind is caused primarily by thinking and talking about the thoughts that are involved in or have caused the depression. Depressive thoughts stir emotions and talking about those thoughts intensifies those emotions. They all work together too, as those emotions intensify, the agitation increases and that drives the depressive thoughts to become even more overwhelming. That cycle continues and increases in intensity as you continue thinking or talking about it. All of it feeds the condition, the confusion becomes deeper and the agitation becomes more severe.

These are some of the reasons, but not the only reasons, why continuous thinking and talking will only make the condition worse. There are other dynamics of the mind and thoughts that are involved and they will be explained in this book.

Peace of mind is not found in thoughts, words and concepts. The very definition of peace is no disturbance or conflict. Peace means tranquility, quiet. Peace of mind is beyond thinking and beyond concept; it is a sustained simple quiet and tranquil condition that happens outside of thinking. When the thoughts that you think bring stress into your mind there is never going to be any peace.

It is unreasonable to assume that any method of thinking and talking will ever solve depressive mental conditions because the entire condition is in and because of the thoughts. Therefore the only way to overcome and heal from depression is to stop thinking the thoughts that cause it and sustain it.

Stopping the thoughts method of dealing with the issues relating to depression is diametrically opposite to everything used, taught and thought in psychology. Once considered, it doesn't take a genius to figure out that thinking and talking about your depression could and would only make it worse. If the problem is in your thoughts, how can you expect that more thinking and talking about it would ever make it go away?

The bases or root of depression and the maladies associated with it is in our conscious thoughts and will continue as we keep thinking and talking about it.

A method of stopping the thoughts is needed. It needs to be understood that stopping to think and talk about the thoughts that have become so overwhelming and intrusive is the key to mental and emotional and spiritual health and healing.

As you think and talk about the thoughts, you are feeding them and making them stronger and more imbedded in your mind.

Refusing to think and talk about the things you have gone over hundreds of times before in your mind and with your words is not suppressing them, it is just a conscious decision to let go of them and refuse to think them anymore.

This book is about learning what is really going on in your mind and thoughts. It is about what really happened to you, how you came to be depressed and what you are doing that continues to feed the overwhelming and intrusive thoughts that you can't stop yourself from thinking. This work explains it all in a comprehensive and reasonable way and in a way that anyone can understand.

Even more importantly it teaches you how to stop thinking the thoughts. How to enable yourself to be able to refuse the thoughts a place in your mind and thought processes. When we are depressed we instinctively know that if we could just stop the thoughts, everything would be fine. That instinct is true and you will come to understand how and why it is true by reading and studying the principles explained in this book. With that knowledge you will come to understand why being still and stopping the thoughts is the process that cures depression.

To make yourself still and stop thinking the thoughts is not suppressing them, it is just a conscious decision to let go of them and refuse to think them anymore.

"No problem can be solved from the same level of consciousness that created it."

Albert Einstein

You can't use your thinking and your mind to figure out or cure what's going on in your thinking and your mind!

Doug Zaccanelli

The Counterproductive Results
of Continuous Therapy

Therapy is good so far as it is used correctly and is appropriate for the condition that it is treating. Counseling an individual can bring about positive change both socially and psychologically. However, whenever the condition is brought about by depression, there comes a time when you need to stop thinking and talking about it. Whenever you are thinking or talking about the problems of depression or conditions associated with it you are perpetuating them.

Psychoanalysis and therapy have an effect and talking about your issues is helpful to a point, but there comes a point in the healing process when you need to let it go in order to continue healing. If you do not and you continue with thinking and talking about it constantly, you not only continue to perpetuate but even to magnify the problem. How can you expect to continually think and talk about the problem all of the time and expect it to ever go away? As you continue that approach, you will find yourself just drawn deeper into the mire and confusion of mind and the overwhelmingly intrusive and destructive thoughts within it.

Even many good intentioned coping mechanisms become counter-productive. Such as when you are trying to avoid those negative and destructive thoughts by focusing your mind on a different, more positive thought, you are still feeding the same mental condition you are trying to avoid. As you are trying to switch your attention to a positive thought in order to avoid its negative counterpart is still feeding the same fundamental condition because it is all one thing, your mind and your thoughts are all connected. Thinking of some seemingly opposite thing in an effort to change thoughts or behavior is feeding the same primary thing, an out of control mind and the thoughts within it!

When you are trying to be mindful or trying to relax and calm yourself by meditating, going to your "happy place", visualizing or even doing something like chanting the word ONE or OM, or any of a multitude of other therapies that are contrived and conceptualized by men, including the multitude of psychological therapies rooted in Freudian theory, you are all of the time using the same mental processes, functions and facilities that the problem is in.

All of these methods continue to feed and sustain the problem. All of these methods may seem to have some effect but they will not solve the underlying problem. Using these methods makes it a certainty that you will eventually find yourself back where you started looking for another coping mechanism.

You can be sure that whenever you are talking or thinking about the problem or doing any one of the things just mentioned in an effort to overcome depression, you are just directing sustaining energy into the root, cause and structure of the problem. How can you expect to overcome your affliction using the same facilities that are afflicted?

Whether you know it or not or believe it or not does not matter, the reality is that you are continuously self-involved in self-creating the life that you are living through and because of the thoughts that you think.

Because it is All Thought

Your own thoughts rule, they are the most influential and powerful thing in your life. Your thoughts are the reason you are who you are and what you have become in life. The overwhelming reason you are where you are in your life is because of the thoughts that you think, moment to moment and day to day.

Whether your thoughts are predominantly good and positive or predominantly destructive and negative, the thoughts that you think rule your present life and are developing the life you will have going forward into your future. Your own thoughts that you think every day and moment to moment are developing and influencing everything in your life and everything in your life experience. Your thoughts are in most ways the only real influence because no matter what happens to you, it is how you perceive and think about it that is the real influence. That seemingly weak and ineffectual thought that is fluttering through your head at this moment in time is a powerful force in building you or damaging you and every single thing going on in your life. It is also the sole reason that you are prosperous or broke, emotionally and psychologically stable or a basket case, a great person to be around or a person to avoid. It is only because of your thoughts that you are happy or miserable. Every single thought you have is another brick in the wall of the life you are building, whether it be a castle or a miserable little shack.

It is all the thoughts that you are thinking day to day and

moment to moment that is the entire cause of your condition. Whether that condition is extreme happiness, success, and a life worth living or depression, failure and dissatisfaction of where and what you and your life has become. All of it, everything, depends on your thoughts and it is only your thoughts.

The reality is that it is not some unconscious memory or situation going on far below the surface in what people call your subconscious that is causing your depression or any of the other conditions associated with depression. It is not some unconscious or buried memories or long forgotten thing that you haven't dealt with yet that is causing the problems either.

Even the things going on around you or happening to you may seem to be the cause of some of the problems you are having, but it is more because of the way that you think about those things that is the major issue. The problem lies in the thoughts you have about those things that affect you more than anything else.

It is very simply the thoughts that you keep thinking every day that continues to exacerbate and escalate the problem. It is not because you got beat up every day in the first grade or you were molested at the age of nine or your mother didn't breast feed you long enough. Many of us have been through serious and overwhelmingly traumatic experiences and still have gone on to a happy and productive life.

You will <u>never</u> think, talk, therapy, meditate, medicate or sleep your depression away!

The overwhelming cause of your depression and misery is the thoughts that you are constantly thinking. It is in those thoughts that you can't let go of, or refuse to let go of, that contain or bring with them the pain and stress you are experiencing. Those are the thoughts you have to let go of and refuse them a place in your mind. Only then will you have relief from that stress and pain.

To move on you must come to the understanding and to know that the thoughts that are passing through your mind right now at this moment in time is the cause of your depression, your unhappiness and every fear and doubt that you have about yourself and what you are experiencing in life. That is the truth of what is going on, that is the reality that you need to understand and accept in order to move on.

To move on you must know that counter to what many practice and believe, you will not change your thoughts or the situation they cause in your life by thinking and talking about them. In fact, the more you think the thoughts or talk about them the worse it will get.

Sanity, mental stability and underlying happiness in life depend almost entirely on your conscious thoughts. All that you aspire to be, all that you seek in life in regards to happiness, peace of mind and emotional stability depends upon your conscious, everyday thoughts. Just as in goal setting, you are in essence, thinking the things that you want into being, your depression or other conditions you experience come about because of the thoughts that you have. In depression you are literally thinking the things that you don't want into being because you can't stop thinking or talking about them.

Your happiness depends upon you having good thoughts that you think without effort, every day, day in and day out. Your happiness depends upon having good, healthy, positive thoughts about yourself, the world around you and your place within it. Healthy thoughts need to dominate your thinking every day in order for you to be happy.

Our happiness depends very little upon our circumstances or the things that are happening to us and around us. We are happy only if we chose to be happy and it is essential to our happiness that we have control of what we allow ourselves to think. Even when "stuff" happens which it inevitably does, we have to control our thinking and what we allow to pass through our mind. We need to be confident in our thoughts and feelings, to know that they are true and real and normal. When the thoughts that we have and our thinking is right, everything else in our life tends to fall into place. That doesn't mean our life becomes perfect, it just means that we become able to deal confidently with everything life throws at us and still have a degree of happiness and peace of mind in spite of our troubles!

When our thoughts are upon the business of living instead of fighting intrusive thoughts and feelings and wondering what is wrong with us all of the time, then we know that our thinking is healthy and normal and we have our life back.

The power to get control of your thoughts and mind begins with having correct knowledge of what is really going on in your head.

Lunch with a Friend

Some years ago my friend and I were eating lunch together one afternoon. As usual the conversation was light and meaningless because, as usual, we spent most of the time more or less mocking each other, not maliciously but in a spirit of friendship. Then it turned serious. My friend, out of the blue, told me that he had been considering suicide for months now and that he had come to the point where he was going to go ahead and do it.

We are good friends but not necessarily close enough that I really knew what was going on with him in his day to day life, we just got together for lunch now and then to catch up. At first I thought he was about to tell me a punch line but then I began to realize that he was serious.

He started telling me that he had been seeing a therapist but, in spite of therapy and other things he has tried, the intrusiveness and uncontrollability of the thoughts he was having just kept getting worse. He went on about how miserable he was and how he couldn't, or didn't want to deal with it anymore. He had come to the conclusion that he was just going to end it the only way that he knew how. He was choosing the way that too many people end up having to choose.

This was not the first time that I had been surprised by somebody in this way but I was very surprised by him because I knew how very strong and confident he was in everything. His candor, in telling me what was going on with him, may have saved his life. He had no idea that I knew how to deal with this type of problem. That I had, over the years, showed many people how to deal with destructive and intrusive thoughts and to heal themselves from depression.

I asked him if he would hold off on his plans for at least two weeks and do exactly what I told him to do. He thought that I was kidding so I had to tell him that I was serious. I also gave him a promise that if he did what I was about to teach him, not only would he feel better in just a few days, but that within a week or two of steady practice he would come to realize that this practice would enable him to heal himself of his depression. I also promised him that because of what he was about to learn he would never have to go through depression again.

I began to teach him the things that are talked about in this book.

Knowledge of what is really happening in his head and the little exercise I was going to teach him would give him all of the power that he needed to take back control of his mind and his thoughts and his life. The power to take back control lies in having correct knowledge of what is really going on in your head and then using that knowledge in a practical and effective way. The practical and effective thing to do is to stop thinking the thoughts because it is the thoughts that are the problem. It takes a little practice to be able to stop the thoughts but it becomes possible with the method that is taught here.

Thoughts may become intense and seem to attack at first because you are denying them the attention they need to exist.

My friend agreed to hold off on his plans for a while, of course, and he agreed to listen to what I was about to teach him. And then to practice the mental exercise I was going to show him how to do.

I began teaching him by telling him what was really going on in his head. I started by explaining some basic and simple things about the mind and thoughts. I explained how thoughts and mind interact with each other in the mental processes. How thoughts are presented to our consciousness in the process of thinking. How thoughts are fed, strengthened and perpetuated as we think them and how they can become intrusive and out of control because of it.

I explained to him why he could not overcome his intrusive thoughts by thinking and talking about them. I explained why therapy, drugs, meditation and mindfulness have little to no positive effect. In fact I said that all of these psychological practices and methods only exacerbate problems with depression. We reasoned together that as he continued to talk about and to think the thoughts, that he was in fact feeding them.

I taught him that by practicing a simple little exercise in mental self-discipline that he could learn how to stop thinking those thoughts.

Finally I taught him how to be still and stop his thoughts.

I also cautioned him that the intrusive thoughts may become intense for a day or two because of his denying them his attention. They may become intense and even attack when he refuses to think them. I told him that it would be best to treat them like white noise for awhile, like the neighbors went to work and left their television on real loud. Even though you can hear it through the wall, you would not sit there and listen to it. That is the way to treat the intrusive thoughts, just ignore them as much as you can and get on with your day. Their attack will only last a short time because as they lose your attention, they are losing their food source. They cannot exist without your thinking them!

After that we parted, he went back to work and so did I. Two days later I called him to check his progress, he picked up the phone and I said," Hey"? In a much stressed out voice he said, "Doug, the thoughts are getting worse. I answered, "didn't I tell you that it might get worse for a couple of days"? Apprehensively he said, "yeah". "What does the thoughts getting worse mean"? I asked him. "Well according to you, it means that it's working". "And what do you think you ought to do about it" I asked. He said, "I think I am going to keep practicing the exercise".

He called me about ten days later and kidded with me when he asked me where he should send the check, I said, "no charge my friend".

You may need to treat those thoughts like white noise for the next few days.

Recovery is because of three things.

- The first is becoming knowledgeable of the true nature of thoughts, how they develop and what sustains them and makes them so intrusive.
- Second, knowing that when you stop thinking the thoughts and talking about them, you stop feeding them and sustaining them and they stop being intrusive and begin to dissipate.
- Third, by using a proven method of being still you will be able to stop thinking and feeding the thoughts and that diminishes their power to be intrusive.

Through regular practice of that little exercise my friend quickly learned to take back control of what was going on in his mind because the exercise is an exercise in controlling your attention. The practice enabled him to take his attention away from unwanted thoughts and feelings in a way that they quickly lost their power and place in his mind. By exercising a little discipline he quickly learned how to stop thinking the thoughts that bothered him.

How many times have we wanted to make all of the thoughts in our head just stop! Learning how to stop the thoughts is what is taught here, the simple little exercise I call Being Still is a method of regaining control and stopping the thoughts, it is about taking our life back in a few short days, not months or years, but in just days!

Instead of constantly thinking and talking about his thoughts, he learned how to stop thinking them. He learned that he needed to stop thinking and talking about the thoughts he was having because talking about and thinking them just magnified them and made them stronger and more dominant in his mind.

By exercising a little mental discipline my friend quickly learned how to stop thinking the thoughts that bothered him.

The thoughts that are fluttering
through your mind at this moment
are affecting you and your life in more
ways than you can ever imagine.

The power to change is all in where you place your attention!

Those seemingly powerless and insignificant things that we call thoughts that are fluttering through your mind at this moment in time are designing, creating and becoming the very substance of your life. And they can only exist there because you think them. As they are passing through your mind and you are allowing yourself to give them your attention, you are feeding them. You will sometimes ask, where do the thought come from and what came first the thought or your attention to it? It is not important to consider that question at this time, what is important is knowing how and why it is that if you deny that thought your attention it cannot exist anymore. The reason it appeared isn't as important as knowing that the reason it keeps coming back is because you give it some attention by thinking it.

Whatever your condition is, whether you are happy or depressed, have PTSD, thoughts of suicide, even bi-polar condition or any of the other mental afflictions people face, the key and solution to real healing is by changing the thoughts that you think. But the "catch 22" reality is that you cannot change your thoughts by simply thinking about it or talking about it.

You must gain control of what you allow yourself to think by controlling what thoughts you give your attention to. Initially the only real control you have in your mind is your attention.

The only reason that thought
exists, is because you keep
allowing yourself to think it

That thought that you are thinking is
a thing of substance that accumulates
more substance as you think it.
And every time you think it, it
gathers more substance.

Where your attention goes energy flows!

Your attention is the key. Initially, it is nearly impossible to control your mind or the thoughts that pass through it, but you can control your attention. When thoughts are denied your attention they lose their power to be. Thoughts gain the power to exist by and through the attention you give to them, and they can become overwhelming and intrusive only from the attention that you give to them.

You can learn how to control your attention. Once you have control of your attention, you will be able to take your attention away from the thoughts that you don't want to think and that alone will bring about significant changes in your life.

Once you become able to refuse to give your attention to the intrusive and damaging thoughts you have been thinking, you have effective control of your mind and your thoughts. In the process you will learn how to stop any and all of your thoughts, effectively being able to remove the energy the uncontrollable and intrusive thoughts need to exist. You will effectively change the entire direction of your life by changing the thoughts that you allow your attention.

It is essential to your mental, emotional and spiritual health and your happiness that you become able to control your mind and all of your mental processes. And you do all of this by learning to control your attention because, remember that where your attention goes sustaining mental energy flows.

Your attention directs the flow of mental energy into the thoughts. That mental energy is what creates and sustains each one of your thoughts. Whether that thought is creating or destroying you, it is only the energy you are feeding into it by thinking it that matters. You must learn to choose the thoughts that you give your attention to.

Thoughts are central in life, your thoughts create and sustain everything going on in your life, they are your life, each one of your thoughts is affecting you and your life in more ways than you can ever imagine.

Your attention directs the flow of mental energy into the thoughts as you are thinking them. That mental energy is the substance that creates and sustains those thoughts.

<u>**Weak and insignificant as thoughts seem, it all begins with thought...**</u>

Every word ever said.
Every thing ever conceived, invented and made.
Every piece of furniture, bicycle or car built, every work of architecture.
Every act, every social movement, every revolution, battle plan or peace accord.
Every story told, every piece of art created, every song sung.
Every poem or love song written and every feeling behind them originated in a thought.....

We Really Are What We Think

As stated in the scriptures, "As a man thinketh in his heart so is he," (Proverbs 23:7). Let us take this scriptural statement literally and try not to color or blur the meaning of it by our own mental limitations, prejudices and capacity to fully understand what the Lord meant when he revealed this concept to us. So it follows according to that statement, we must be just that, we are what we think physically, mentally psychologically and spiritually. We are what we think right down to and into our very bones.

Your entire life is a product of the thoughts that you have thought and those thoughts that you now entertain. You are most what you have thought about the most, but even the lesser thoughts have an impact on who and what you have become.

If you are with me so far then you know that when you are depressed or have any conditions like it or associated with it, you are experiencing what happens when too many of your thoughts are negative, self-effacing and self-degrading and they have been that way for far too long a time. If you and your life is built by your thoughts, all that you think now and everything that you have ever thought is a part of who and what you are and what you are becoming, period.

Some of these concepts can be as subtle as a thought itself but reason bears them out to be true.

We are fools if we think that some of our thoughts are meaningless and ineffective in shaping us and our life. Every little thought that we have has meaning and influence in our lives.

We may want to think that only our great thoughts are the ones that have effect in our life and the ones in between, the ones we think when we are not really paying attention to our thoughts, are ineffective and meaningless.

While it is true that the thoughts that we think the most and put a lot of energy and focus into are a greater influence in our lives and in determining who and what we are, it should follow also that if the big ones affect us then the little ones will also have some effect. So then you should ask yourself, how damaging are those intrusive thoughts that I am thinking right now, given that every single one of my thoughts has an effect in my life.

Think of how those intrusive and overwhelming thoughts are ruining everything in your life. In fact at this point, if you are depressed, you really do not have a life, at least not a life that you can call worth living. But don't worry or do anything hasty, that condition will soon change because you are coming to understand what is really going on within you, and you will also learn what you can do to correct it.

The things that happen to us and those things going on around us and the things we have witnessed all have an effect on us. But all of those things only affect us by and through the way that we think of them and about them. Everything in our life and in the life we experience is about and because of our thoughts, absolutely EVERYTHING!

"If you *correct your thoughts*, the rest of your life will fall into place"

Lao Tzu, Chinese philosopher

The thoughts you are having at this very moment determines your life. They are creating or destroying your happiness. Your thoughts are creating the substance of your entire life. Every moment of your life is spent thinking thoughts, your day is filled with them. They determine everything about your life and not only what your life is like now but what it will be in the future. What you are thinking at this very moment affects you now, it will affect you in ten minutes, in two hours and in five and in ten years. Your life, order, sanity and happiness all depends on how and what you think about, and what you allow to pass through your mind. You are constantly becoming what you are thinking and your thoughts are shaping and defining you and the life you are experiencing. And this is a self-perpetuating condition because the thoughts that you have now leads to the next thought which has the seed of the next thought within it and it just goes on and on.

You and your life is created and built by your thoughts. All that you think now and everything that you have ever thought is a part of who and what you are and what you are becoming.

"No one saves us but ourselves.
No one can and no one may.
We ourselves must walk the path."

Buddha

How Will It Ever Go Away?

If you spend so much of your day thinking and talking about your problem with depression, how can you expect it to ever go away?

How many times have you said to yourself, "if I could somehow just stop thinking these thoughts that everything would be fine"? That assumption is correct, because it is in fact those conscious ever present thoughts that are causing your depression and the unhappiness, misery, confusion and hopelessness you are feeling.

It is those depressive thoughts that are getting in the way of everything else in your life.

Many have tried to change their thoughts and have had limited success. Many of us have said to ourselves, "I am going to start thinking positive." Perhaps we were determined and said I am going to think positive from now on. Only to find ourselves, within a moment or two, thinking the same old thoughts we have been fighting all along. Sound familiar? It has been observed that every time we take a breath we have another thought come into our mind. So if we observe and wonder how quickly we can go from having a firm resolve to start thinking positive and to then falling right back into the same old pattern of thinking, it can be measured by the length of only one or two breaths.

Thoughts cannot be merely replaced by different or newer and unfamiliar thoughts; they are there and have a place in your mind. You have thought those thoughts many, many times and the attention you have given them has given them strength and substance and they are embedded in your mind. To just try and replace them with new unfamiliar thoughts is almost like trying to replace your children with different ones. Your own children will just keep coming back and clinging to you and the new ones that you have tried to adopt will not stay with you because they have no place.

To really change your thoughts and really affect the mind set or thought pattern that you are in, you have to weaken it. The only way to weaken the pattern is to stop thinking the thoughts within it. That not only weakens the pattern but at the same time it breaks down the thoughts within it. When you stop thinking them it diminishes their power to even exist and in a short time removes them. This is what happens in the course of healing when you stop thinking or refuse to think the thoughts. Not only are the intrusive thoughts that plague you weakened and lose their hold upon your mind, but true and constructive thoughts will start to flood back in.

Although this whole process will take a little time, there are some immediate effects that you will experience. Your mind will be a calmer and clearer. Because you refuse to think the thoughts, you will stop having to deal with the stress they bring with them into your life. Because of less stress in your life, your sleep will improve.

Being able to sleep is one of the first results and proof positive that practice of this exercise brings positive results.

Many times we are deceived by the seeming complexity of a problem into thinking that the solution could not be simple. At the same time we find that the most sophisticated solutions to many problems are often quite simple.

STOP THINKING AND TALKING ABOUT IT!

Whatever you think and talk about, you are inadvertently feeding.

Stop Thinking and Talking About The Thoughts!

Because of these conditions, because you cannot think or talk or therapy, medicate or meditate your way out of these conditions then what can be done?

Not any of the ways invented or contrived by men have produced a cure for depression or any of the conditions associated with it. Every destructive mental condition is rooted in depression except those that are mental conditions resulting from birth defects, injury or physical deficiencies. Even substance abuse is initially rooted in depression and will be affected by stopping the thoughts. Any time spent practicing the discipline of Being Still will greatly help any condition.

Being Still is healing in the Lords way, Gods way. In the Old Testament of The King James Bible, Psalms 46:10, He tells us to "be still and know that I am god". Be still, sit still, don't move, be silent and be still in body and mind and spirit is the Lords prescription for a lot of things and one of them is overcoming depression. Most especially be still in your mind, stop the thoughts and hold the mind still or blank as much as you are able to for just a few minutes a day.

Again "be still and know" is a key to healing. In this very short verse the Lord has given us a simple solution to most mental, emotional and spiritual problems.

Of the many people I have taught to be still over many years of teaching it, many of whom were seriously depressed, some even on the verge of suicide, I have never had anyone come to me and say, "it didn't work for me". To be still is wise and universal counsel because it is the balm that heals everybody mentally, emotionally and spiritually.

Even those with the most long term and severe depression can use this method to overcome their problem. This practice will take effort, nothing is free, but over time most, if not all, of your problems with depression will go away. Consistent practice of this method bears significant results, but even a few efforts will have an effect. This method has proven itself time and time again in overcoming stress, depression and the other mental and emotional disorders associated with depression.

It is universally effective in overcoming these conditions because the root of all mental and emotional problems is depression. The root of depression is in the thoughts that you think. Every condition, including depression, post-partum depression, bi-polar, OCD, PTSD and the emotional issues that accompany them is because of thoughts.

Learning how to stop thinking the thoughts is central to this discipline. Learning how to stop thinking the thoughts and letting them go is essential to healing. You will not get better if you continue to hold onto and not let go of the destructive things in your life, forgiveness of yourself and others is essential to healing.

Being Still

is not psychology,
it is not talking about it,
it is not trying to alter behavior or thoughts or thinking positive,
it is not analysis,
it is not hypnosis,
it is not mindfulness,
it is not self-talk,
it is not thinking about it,
it is not meditation because that is thinking also!
It is not going to your happy place, chanting, relaxing or visualizing,
Being Still *is* non-talking, non-thinking, non-conceptualizing,
It is taking control of your attention and holding everything still, body, mind and spirit.
The result of consistent practice of the exercise of being still is that it calms and quiets the mind and the thoughts…that is how and why it works.

This is not Meditation.

When we are Being Still we are not trying to go to our happy place or thinking about relaxing or trying to feel inner peace. All of these methods involve thinking and conceptualizing, the very thing we are trying not to do.

Being Still is training the mind, it takes discipline, pro-active structured mental discipline. This is a method of controlling your attention and taking it away from thoughts and the thinking process. Your attention is the key, when you refuse to give your attention to the thoughts that come into your mind, you are effectively interrupting or stopping the flow of mental energy into them.

In doing this exercise you are trying to hold your mind and your mental processes still. Just a moment or two of holding the mind and thinking processes still, when done consistently, has a calming and healing effect. When stopping the flow of thoughts it interrupts the natural flow of the mental process. This also brings release from stress because it is the thoughts that bring the stress into the mind with them.

That is why Being Still is non-thinking and non-conceptualizing, it is a concentrated, conscious effort to stop and still all mental activity.

The results of doing this will bring order and structure to the mind, clear thinking instead of confusion, peace instead of fears, confidence instead of doubt, happiness instead of misery.

Sanity, confidence, emotional stability, understanding and clearness of thinking will come to those that practice Being Still regularly.

The regular practice of Being Still will relieve the stress and heal the depressed. No other exercise or discipline conceived by men can equal the unsearchable wisdom and power of the simple little God given exercise that is being still and letting go of the thoughts.

When the Lord tells us, "to be still", He is revealing to us a process of knowing Him better, as a part of this natural process we will overcome and be healed of our mental and emotional afflictions. Through regular practice we will have a deeper spiritual experience as well. He knows all of our struggles and those things in life that we cannot think our way out of so He provided a way that is in many ways beyond the understanding of men. In doing this method you will learn that there is an experience that is higher than the one you are living on. Long term practice of Being Still will bring an inner peace that can't be explained, it can only be experienced.

This is a proactive, structured mental exercise that takes focused, conscious and aggressive mental effort.

Peace of mind does not come from thinking.

The Art of Being Still

Being Still begins with controlled breathing. Remember that the key to controlling your mind and your thoughts is in where you place your attention. Use your breath to calm yourself and as a point to focus your attention on.

Breath is central to life and it is the physical connection to the mind and the mental process. Evidence of this connection is demonstrated by observing how a person that is losing control and becoming upset will breathe rapid and shallow, while a person that is relaxed or focused will breathe slow and even. Our thoughts, mind and mental state affects our breathing. That connection travels both ways and it is because of this connection between breath and mind that we are able to affect our mind and mental state through our breathing.

By controlling and slowing our breathing we find that it will help us to calm, clear and still our mind and the thoughts that we think. It is done by focusing all of our attention on our breathing, slowing it and letting go of and refusing to think the thoughts that come into our mind as we practice the exercise. By focusing all of our attention on our breathing and controlling it, we become better able to refuse to give those intrusive type thoughts a place in our mind. The effect of doing this process or discipline is that we become increasingly able to deny thoughts our attention.

One of the dynamics of mind and thought is that certain

thoughts, thoughts such as lies and fantasy, cannot exist unless we think them. When we are thinking the thought we are giving our attention to it. That attention directs the flow of mental energy into it, which feeds the thought with sustaining mental energy. Where our attention goes, mental energy flows. Our attention is what an intrusive thought seeks.

Certain types of thoughts, thoughts that are not based in reality, are literally absorbing mental energy from us as we think them. They keep coming back because they are seeking our attention and the mental energy our attention carries with it. That is how and why they become intrusive and overwhelming. Those types of thoughts cannot exist without our attention. Hence untrue thoughts cannot exist unless we think them. When we refuse to give those thoughts our attention we are diminishing their power to exist. At the same time we are releasing the stress the thoughts bring with them. It is the thoughts that cause or bring stress into your life.

When it comes to stress, it is not so much what happens, but how you take it in and deal with it or don't deal with it that causes the stress. So when you refuse the thought you are refusing the stress it carries with it. Stress and worry depletes and wastes energy needed to deal with situations. When practicing Being Still we let go of it for now and will deal with it when its time.

That is why you will be somewhat relaxed and feel lighter of mind and spirit immediately after you practice the exercise.

Denying those thoughts a place in your mind also denies the stress that those thoughts bring with them into your life.

How I still my thoughts.

- I sit up straight with my spine in align, not stiff or rigid but good posture. Or I lay flat on the floor. I need to be able to comfortably take in a full breath of air. Using good posture and this breathing will relax and release much of the tension that is in my back and neck. My spine will actually straighten as I do this.
- I kick all of the air out of my lungs. Then I breathe in through the nose and out through the mouth. Slow and purposeful. I take at least twice as long to exhale as it did to inhale. I find that the longer it takes to exhale the better; I have better control of my attention as I exhale.
- I concentrate on my breathing, I breathe slow. I never hold my breath.
- My attention will start to wander as it follows a thought; I bring it back to my breathing and hold it there. As my attention wanders again, I just keep bringing it back to my breathing. I will have to constantly bring my attention back to my breathing. It is natural for my attention to want to follow a thought. In doing this exercise I am interrupting the natural flow of the mental processes. I have been practicing this for forty plus years and I still have to willfully hold my attention on my breathing.

- After a few minutes of concentrating on my breathing I practice stilling the mind. I still the mind by focusing all my attention on my breath as I inhale, taking a full breath. Then as I exhale, I exhale slow and purposeful, controlling the expiration of breath. I don't allow any thoughts in, I hold my mind blank. I accomplish this by willful control of my attention in much the same way that I am controlling my breathing. I don't let my breath just go out, I control it. I do the same with my attention. I don't let it go; I use my will to control it. I seat all of my conscious attention on my breath and hold it there; I continually practice holding my mind blank on long slow controlled exhales. I refuse any and all thoughts a place in my mind!

- My mind and thoughts are continually trying to distract me during this practice. The aim and purpose for these few minutes are, above all else, to control my attention and be still! I find I have the most power and control over my mind and my thoughts as I exhale. As I exhale I practice holding my mind blank. I keep everything still as I slowly and purposely let my breath out and I hold my mind blank.

After at least 8 minutes. Notice how you feel, observe the differences in your mind and thoughts right after you do this exercise. After more than 40 years of teaching this method, I am still amazed at the effects it has on the people who practice it. If you do this you will experience an immediate change for the better in your mental, emotional and spiritual life. You will become more relaxed and you will even sleep better. In fact one of the first effects of practicing Being Still is that it will help you to sleep. A good night sleep is essential in the fight to overcome depression.

The peace and lightness of mind you
feel right after practice will increase
in duration and degree over time
as you consistently practice.

Being Still is a Refuge and the Balm that heals!

Actually, by focusing your attention on your breathing you will find refuge, it is where you can go to escape the thoughts that you do not want to think or act on. When the overwhelming and intrusive thoughts come in, you can go to your breathing and focus your attention on your breath coming in and going out and ignoring everything else going on within you and around you. In the beginning it may not be easy and at other times it will seem to be a struggle, but I assure you that if you keep doing it you will see results. Treating those thoughts like white noise by refusing to give them any of your attention will starve them out. You should practice doing that as you go about your day when you feel negative or stressful thoughts try to seep in.

Stilling and blanking the mind is the healing balm, as you practice holding your mind blank in a structured and regular practice, you will become healed because you are interrupting the flow and denying the thoughts the attention that they need. At the same time this process is forcing the mind to calm and as it calms it will clear.

You have experienced to some degree the extreme outer edge of where your mind with uncontrolled thoughts can take you. As you have learned in the previous pages it is the thoughts that take you there, whether you just allow yourself to think your way there or you have fought tooth and nail, trying to figure it all out on the way, the result has been the same. So what is left if all of that thinking, talking, meditating, therapy, mindfulness, medicating and maybe even praying didn't seem to work for you?

Being Still takes daily effort, but with that daily effort you will realize immediate benefits, you will feel some degree of immediate peace and a lighter mind and spirit during and immediately after practicing. That peace and lightness of mind will increase in duration and degree over time as you consistently practice.

On the path to healing, Being Still will become something that you can hold onto. It becomes a part of your day, the place that you go to every morning and evening to continue your healing process and it will also be a place to go to when you are feeling low. I encourage you to have a spot in your home where you practice, and if you practice at the same time and in the same place every day, that place will soon become a sanctuary. But remember that it doesn't matter where you are or what is going on at any given time, Being Still is a refuge for you to go to when you feel yourself becoming stressed or overwhelmed. You can practice Being Still on the beach or on the bus, nobody will know that you are practicing as you sit quietly and breathe.

In the beginning do this practice for at least 8 minutes or longer every day, twice a day or more is best. The results are immediate, within a few days after you start to practice Being Still you will notice that you will get to sleep easier and your sleep will be longer and deeper. Everybody progresses at a different rate according to the length of time they practice, but the effects are sure and will continue to reveal themselves over time. You will be amazed!

Be assured, as you practice the exercise, even holding your mind still for a moment or two will have a profound effect on your mental, emotional and spiritual health.

Stillness comes to us in short moments at first. And if we spend the time it takes, the moments lengthen and the quiet becomes delicious to our souls.

Everything originates in thought;
learn to control your thoughts
and you can do anything.

Our Conscious and Intelligent Spirit

The definition of consciousness is; that part of us that is intelligent and conscious of ourselves as individual and separate from the world. Consciousness is that part of us that is our spirit. Consciousness is our conscious and intelligent spirit. I wish to clarify and define consciousness to avoid being vague or misunderstood. When I speak of consciousness I am meaning your conscious intelligent spirit and vice versa.

The part of you that science and psychology ignores is the most important part of you and, perhaps, the least understood. The part of you that is suffering because of your depression, the part of you that is happy or miserable because of your condition is your spirit, your conscious and intelligent spirit.

I want to explain the relationship between your conscious intelligent spirit and your mind and the thoughts within your mind. Understanding this relationship is extremely important because it explains how you are designed and made.

You are conscious and intelligent, the part of you that is conscious and intelligent is your spirit and that is a part of you that is separate from your mind. Your mind, your thoughts and that conscious intelligent part of you are all separate, each with its own purpose and design. These three parts each take part in the mental process and each of them has their own separate purpose and function. Your conscious and intelligent spirit is the most significant and important of these three.

My spirit is a part of me just as your spirit is a part of you. Our spirits are the conscious and intelligent part of us, the life force, that part of us that is living and breathing and occupying our body. Your conscious and intelligent spirit is the part of you that is affected by your living experience, including the things that are going on in your mind.

Your spirit is that part of you that makes decisions and choices and feels the effects of those decisions and choices. It feels the experience you are having in life, it is the part of you that feels the benefits and suffers the wrongs of whatever happens to you in your life.

Individual conscious intelligence is the first principle of our existence. Your conscious intelligence is light, it is the life force, it is that infinite and immortal thing we call our spirit, it is the witness to life and it is the part of you that enjoys the experiences of life and living. Your conscious and intelligent spirit is who you are, what you are, it is that part of you that loves another and has the experience and the feelings that are associated with happiness or misery, fulfillment or emptiness. Your conscious intelligent spirit is that quality within you that is learning and progressing and making right or wrong choices about life and the business of living.

The relationship between your conscious intelligence and your mind will help you to understand how depression and emotional turmoil develops and continues to affect you and will continue because of what you are probably doing as you are trying to deal with it.

The life within you is conscious
and intelligent, that intelligence is
light and that light is infinite.

"That which is of God is light; and he that
receiveth light, and continueth in god,
receiveth more light; and that light groweth
brighter and brighter until the perfect day."

Verse 50:25 of the Book of Doctrine & Covenance

I like to use my pond as a metaphor to help you to understand what is really going on within you. This will illustrate the difference between your conscious and intelligent spirit and your mind and how the relationship they have with each other works.

My favorite place to walk takes me down a wooded path deep into the woods and to the banks of a beautiful and remote woodland pond. It's not very deep as I can see the bottom and there are plenty of reeds and cattails at its shores. There are a few large moss covered rocks on its banks which provide a few good places to sit.

Upon the water, dragonfly's dart and hover and there are some lily pads that flower in the summer. Turtles and frogs are in residence, large and small, swimming around in it.

On a clear day when the wind is calm and there isn't a lot of disturbance in the pond I can see the bottom. As I walk toward the water, I can see the clouds of dust trailing behind the frogs skimming along the bottom as they dart away from the edge that I approach. As they skim along the bottom I see little trails of dust from the muck their passing stirs up, almost like the vapor trails of a supersonic jet. It is fun to watch.

On a cloudy, windy and rainy day the muck and water of the pond gets churned up and I cannot see the frogs or their trails and I don't know, but I assume that they can't see me either.

Let me use my pond to illustrate the relationship between your conscious intelligent spirit and your mind. Now in this illustration, the part of your being that is you, your conscious intelligent spirit or consciousness is laying at the bottom of the pond looking up through the water into the day. The water in that pond represents your mind in this example and your spirit, your conscious intelligent spirit uses the water/mind as a lens to perceive the world through.

When the water/mind is calm and clear, you can see the day as it is. As you look up through the calm and clear water you can see the sun shining and the trees swaying, the blue sky and the puffy clouds rolling by. You can see the birds as they fly over and even the dragonfly's as they hover and dart over the surface, you see all these things as they truly are in reality. All the things in the world around you, you perceive in the way they are, unclouded, uncolored, undistorted through the calm, clear waters that represent your mind.

Then it starts to sprinkle, those little raindrops cause ripples on the surface of the pond and now what you see through the water/mind is a little distorted. You still can see the sun, the clouds, and the blue sky but there is a little distortion so you cannot make out subtleties such as the dragonfly or water bugs.

Then, as the sprinkle turns to rain the distortion increases, doesn't it? Soon you can only see some of the blue sky and some fuzzy patches of white where the clouds are. You can no longer distinguish the sun though it still gives its light.

Look deep into nature, and then you will understand everything better.

Albert Einstein

Then comes the storm and as the wind picks up the water becomes agitated, further distorting your perceptions.

In time your perceptions have changed from seeing a clear, defined reality in the light of a calm and clear sunny day to distortion and confusion, eventually even darkness if the storm is hard and continues long enough to kick up the muck at the bottom of the pond. Now you are cut off from seeing anything clearly, all of your perceptions have become distorted and you cannot be sure of what is really going on in the world around you.

Not unlike the experiences of life from the minor disappointments, like a summer sprinkle to the storms that we all go through in life, things that happen can unsettle us and interrupt our peace. Our perception and our understanding is affected not only by the storm we are going through but also by the things already going on here within us. All of the negative things we have held onto affect us and they are magnified most in times of stress and difficulty. We will learn that that is why Being Still and letting go of those things and forgiveness of ourselves and others is so important in helping us recover from mental and emotional problems.

The water of the pond represents the substance of mind that acts as the lens that we experience life through. The sun represents light and understanding, clouds and wind and rain represent situations and adversities in life. The muck within the pond represents the negative and unhealthy thoughts, feelings and experiences that we hold onto.

Life is change, sun, rain, clouds, storms and seasons are all a part of nature, in some ways we are a part of nature and like everything else in nature, we and our situations are constantly changing. From the minor disappointments we all have, like when we are in a hurry to get to school or work and the car won't start or we miss our bus, these are like the summer sprinkle, they unsettle us but usually have no lasting effect. Losing our job or our spouse leaving us represents the storms of life and living, all will pass but in the moment we find ourselves in turmoil, barely able to cope. Life is change and our attitude and our ability to deal with the change, to take the blows and let go of it, determines our happiness.

We need to let go of the bad things that have happened, things we have done and things others have done to us. When we do not let go of and truly forgive ourselves and those who trespass against us, it is just baggage that piles up. When we don't let go, or we refuse to let go, we carry those things with us as baggage and we will have to deal with the negative forces that baggage carries with them. These things bring us down and they can get heavier when we are dealing with the adversities in life. Sometimes those things we hold onto are the things that bring on the adversities. We all have things happen in our lives and it is in the way that we deal with them or hold onto them that can poison the mind and weigh it down.

The water of the pond represents your mind which is like the lens that you, as a conscious and intelligent spirit, perceives and experiences life through.

Learn to Let Go of Things.

Just remember always that thoughts are things, unhealthy thoughts and feelings about yourself and others are like heavy baggage, not only do they weigh you down, they will become a destructive force within you and can be the cause of depression and other psychological problems if you hold on and won't let go of them. Just like the muck lying at the bottom of the pond, the unhealthy things that we have held onto are waiting there to be stirred up and darken and cloud our mind. By letting go of them you can minimize or completely take away any lasting or reoccurring affect they can have on you.

There are two seas in the land of Israel, the Sea of Galilee and The Dead Sea. In and around the Sea of Galilee the environment is teeming with life. Water flows into Galilee freely and flows out freely. In Galilee there is a constant never ending flow and renewal of abundant life giving nourishment from the water flowing through it. The Dead Sea and the areas surrounding it are dead; water flows in but does not flow out as it does in Galilee. The flow is dammed, the water stagnates and evaporates and the impurities that are left, kills rather than nourishes everything in its environs.

So much can be learned from simple examples. How damming can holding on to something be in your life?

Begin to let go of the thoughts as you realize you are thinking them while practicing Being Still. Then practice letting go of thoughts while you are out in the day, let go of the anger, the pain, the memory, the fear it brings. Let go of everything because everything you hold onto becomes a part of you.

Letting go is an integral and important part of the healing process. You will find it hard to progress if you refuse to let go of any ill thoughts or feelings that you are holding onto. As your mind calms and thoughts and feelings surface you need to let go of everything, thoughts, fear, anger and any resentment you are holding onto.

Remember, it is the thoughts and your attention to them that is the problem. As you continue to think the same negative and intrusive thoughts while you are trying to figure yourself out, you will inevitably continue in your closed off world of negative self-discussion and continue feeding those thoughts that perpetuate the problems. Letting go is an integral and necessary part of the healing process.

Reason out what is real and true in your life and what will bring lasting happiness to yourself and those people around you. Forgive yourself and others the trespasses. Forgiveness is not weakness, it is strength, you will become a great person if you can learn to let go of all but loving and positive thoughts and feelings about yourself and others. Negative thoughts really are a disease and if you hold on to them they will fester and just become a bigger problem in your life. So let go of all that is negative in your mind and heart. Letting go is part of the healing process. It is always your choice whether to let go of things and there are times when you need to turn the other cheek for your own wellness and peace.

Letting go of thoughts while you are practicing Being Still leads to becoming better able to let go of thoughts and the things they carry with them into your life, even while you are out in your day.

Be still and know, be still and let go.

Let go of that thought, let go of that thinking, let go of that feeling, let go of that fear, let go of that anger. By letting go of everything it gives us back the power of determining what our thoughts will be. By holding our mind still and refusing the thought a place in our mind or willfully letting go of it we are letting go of the feeling and the emotion attached to it. By refusing the thought we are also denying the force and strength of any influence it has in our mind and in our life. That action also diminishes the power and strength of a flawed or incorrect mind-set that we have developed and don't even know that we have.

When Being Still we are letting go of all thoughts, both positive and negative, true and untrue. When we do that we are also letting go of those things that have helped to form our perception of things, and our beliefs. The way we perceive things form the way we believe things are or ought to be. Even when the basis for the perception is wrong or untrue it has still shaped the way that we think and believe. When our perceptions are based on false or untrue information and concepts it becomes somewhat impossible to know reality.

It really does not matter what we believe, what matters is what is true and real. This process helps us to become free of things that we haven't been able to let go of or reason our way through. We are all stunted by thoughts and beliefs we have developed that are incorrect and even harmful to our mental, emotional and spiritual health.

We all have an abundance of flaws in our thinking. Because within our thoughts exist formed concepts which have flaws and misconceptions about ourselves and the world and those around us. These are thoughts and concepts that can be formed based on flawed, incorrect or incomplete information.

Once we can acknowledge that we all have flaws that we need to overcome, who can or will tell us what they are? "why beholdest the mote in thy brothers eye and not the beam that is in thine eye" Matthew 7:3. Can we ourselves or a therapist that we are talking to become so insightful as to identify all of our flaws, even the flaws in our thinking and how they developed or what we can do to correct them? Is anyone that clever?

As we practice regularly the discipline of Being Still, our mind takes on a level of stillness. From this our mind calms and clears and it reveals a lot of things that we could not or would not see before. This is called personal revelation which spawns in us personal growth and inspiration. Knowledge of who we are, inspiration in daily living and correct choices in life brings personal growth in our mental, emotional and spiritual lives.

By refusing the thought our attention we
are also denying the emotional force and the
strength of any influence that thought brings
with it into our mind and into our life.

Being Still is the key, it is the key and the tool, and it is the means to an end. Being Still is the balm that heals. All of the thinking and talking we have done to this point may have helped diagnose and define the problem. But there has to be a point when we let go of it, otherwise it just remains there in front of us. Further discussion only goes to help reinforce the problem(s) and make it stronger and more dominant in our life and makes for more confusion. If we continue to perpetually think about it and talk about it, how can it ever leave us? If we continue to treat our condition in this way, the condition will soon, if it hasn't already, become dominate and control everything in our life.

We, all of us, come to the point when it is time to let go of certain things because we need to for our mental, emotional and spiritual health and that is the real purpose of practicing Being Still. The way to practice Being Still is to interweave within the discipline, the continual practice of letting go. We start by learning to let go of the thoughts as they enter the mind during the practice of Being Still. As we do that we also learn to let go of the feelings and anger and any destructive forces that the thoughts carry with them. In fact we learn to let go of any and all thought good or bad while we are actively practicing Being Still. We should, in wisdom, extend that practice into our daily living and thinking. As we continually let go of the intrusive and destructive thoughts they begin to lose their power to be intrusive and it happens that the feelings, such as anger or resentment that accompany those thoughts lose their influence also.

There comes a time in life when if we do not start to let go of the unhealthy thoughts we are having and the things accompanying them they will begin to define us. Letting go of thoughts is not suppressing them it is merely ceasing to give them our attention.

Another of the healthy benefits of Being Still is as we learn to let go of intrusive and unhealthy thoughts, as we stop dwelling on them, we will start to see them differently. In most cases we will start to understand them correctly. As we calm our minds and let go of them it will also remove the emotions attached to them. That changes our perception of them and usually our concept of them being a problem begins to disintegrate, that allows the problem to either present its own solution or we come to the realization that it is not worth our attention and we are glad to just let it go.

Being Still is healing in the Lords
way, He tells us to, "be still and
know that I am God".

Psalms 46:10
King James Bible

This is the Lords council, He is the master
psychologist. He is telling us that we need
to be still, to stop trying to think, talk
or meditate our way out of depression.

Being Still Accomplishes Many Things

Stopping the thoughts does many things, both during your practice of the discipline and then continues to have ongoing healing benefits afterward. The practice of stopping the thoughts initially causes healing from depression and many other psychological issues associated with it. Regular practice promotes increasing and deeper degrees of self-realization which can only make you stronger on every level and situation in life. As you continue to practice, you will experience positive mental, social and spiritual growth, you will become more self-aware, self-reliant and self-confident. All of the benefits that can be realized are beyond description and most of them can only be experienced, so I urge everyone to continue practicing even after you have cleared your life of the maladies that brought you to the practice.

During and then for some time after each practice its effect immediately calms and clears your mind and thinking. As you continue to practice regularly the calmness continues longer into the day and becomes deeper and more profound.

As you continue to practice consistently, the mind and the thought processes become calmer because as you refuse to think thoughts and practice blanking your mind during those long slow exhales, you are in effect, forcing your mind to calm. As the mind calms it becomes clearer. Just as turbulent waters become calm, they clear and clearer waters reveal everything within them. So a calmer mind enables clearer and correct perceptions of the things going on in your life and experiences.

As your perceptions become clearer you can choose to think only those thoughts that are healthy, judging all things from a calmer and clearer and even higher perspective.

All of these things happen gradually and simultaneously, and they start happening as soon as you begin to practice the exercise for the first time. Your condition starts to improve immediately and continues to improve as you continue to practice.

Right from the first time you practice the exercise you will notice that you are calmer and clearer right at the completion of your daily practice. As days go by and you continue practice you continue to improve. It is not long before you realize that as long as you continue to practice the discipline you will continue to improve and you will gain confidence in knowing that you will never have to deal with problems like this again. Your thoughts soon become centered on the business of living instead of what is wrong with you

Do not look for great spiritual experiences only while you are practicing Being Still, but rather look for a lighter, brighter and higher experience in your day and throughout your life.

THE SCIENCE OF MIND
AND THOUGHT

Correct knowledge and understanding of the true nature of mind and thought and their relationship with your conscious intelligent spirit will give you deeper understanding and help set you free!

Thoughts are Primal

We are conscious and intelligent creators. The conscious and intelligent part of us is the creators and sustainers of the thoughts we think. Thoughts are the beginning of everything that is created, they are primary. Everything ever created or made was preceded by a thought. Some say creation began with a word, which undoubtedly was preceded by a thought. Certainly our own creative process begins with thought. Your thoughts are the designer and creator of everything in your life, they form the substance and the fabric of everything that exists in you, in your life and in your experience.

Thoughts are everything and they affect everything within you and without you and they affect or control almost everything that goes on within your entire environment.

These statements may seem to be a bit overreaching and it may be difficult to comprehend the enormity of what they mean but take a moment and think about it. You have to admit that everything ever said everything that has been written, every act performed, everything that has been invented and made, absolutely everything that is within and without physical creation started with a thought, is thought, or the result of thought. Thoughts are the beginning of everything that is created. We live or exist in a created and creative sphere. Whatever is created and manifested within this sphere, even the situations that exist within it are created and made because of, or out of the thoughts that precede it.

Part of and indeed the beginning of your own creative process is the creation of thought. You are the creator of your own life and experience by and through your thoughts. Your ideas are thoughts that you created and they are things of substance as soon as they are formed in your mind. That thought that exists in your mind is a thing of substance that accumulates more substance as you think it. And every time you think it, it gathers more substance.

Thinking that thought is how and why it has existence and only by thinking it has it the power to become. When it is a thought that is in any way related to yourself, as in the way you view yourself, it is either a thing that is uplifting and building of a great life and experience or it will be a destructive force. If it's a destructive force it will have the potential to become overwhelming and intrusive as you continue to allow yourself to think it. But remember this, the only way that thought can and will exist is because you think it and continue to allow yourself to think it.

That thought that exists in your mind is a thing of substance that accumulates more substance as you think it. And every time you think it, it gathers more substance.

Substance of Thought and Mind

It may be unreasonable at first for you to think of thoughts as a force or substance. We want to continue to think of them as being nothing but weak and ineffectual, without structure, substance or power. The idea of thoughts having any significant power still eludes the reasonable mind because there does not exist any empirical evidence that thoughts have actually become anything. Our mind wants to dismiss anything that cannot produce hard evidence that our senses cannot see, touch and feel.

It is an illusion in nature that the weak and insignificant things in nature only appear that way. Think for a moment of the apparent weakness and insignificance of a drop of water. In fact think about the insignificance and weakness of vapor. You cannot see, touch or barely feel vapor. For the most part you can only see vapor coming out of a tea kettle when it is boiling. Otherwise you cannot see it at all. But at a certain temperature that vapor becomes a drop of water.

That drop of water is a little bit more significant than vapor and you can see it, touch it and feel it. We need many drops of water to maintain life, our own life and the lives of everything we eat. Yet water seems so weak and insignificant.

But what about ice. That vapor is now a thing of substance that has structure, weight and strength, it has now become a thing of substance. Massive substance in fact, imagine the massive size of some icebergs. We only see about a third of the mass of an iceberg above the surface of the water.

I can go on about the wonders of nature and creation, in fact think about or consider vapor which is evaporated water which when it hits a mass of cool air it turns to rain or snow. Sometmes it turns to a lot of rain, even enough rain to fill the ocean. Then that warm ocean water and wind currents create a hurricane which causes a flood, and waves that destroy! Now that vapor or drop of water is not so insignificant is it? In fact that same drop of water is a life giving and sustaining force one moment and then become a terrible destructive force the next.

Life and nature teaches us that the seeming weak things in life are actually the most powerful, while the seemingly strong and powerful things are in fact at the mercy of the weak things. The hardest rock will get wore down and become smooth as the water of a stream runs over and around it, or the wind blows against it.

How weak and powerful, life giving and destructive is the wind? When was the last time that you saw the wind?

It is true that the seemingly weaker things in nature and in creation are in fact the strongest and most powerful! In fact the seemingly weaker and insignificant a thing is, the stronger and more significant it is!

Do you still maintain in your mind that thoughts are not that significant in your life?

Mind is pure energy, mental energy.
Our thoughts create and form that
energy into things of substance.

Thoughts and the Activity of Thinking

We each have our own thoughts that exist in our mind. If you are like most of us, some of those thoughts are true and some of those thoughts are false. Some are clear and defined and some may not be. Some thoughts will seek to dominate your attention, while others are passive and they do not come into your mind unless you call them up by searching in your mind for them. Thoughts such as facts, knowledge and most memories do not come into your mind unless you call on them. Thoughts such as, *my third grade teacher's name was Mrs. Keenen* or *"my spouses birthday is April 10th "*, only come into your mind when you call them up or search in your memory banks for them. Usually a memory comes to mind when it is triggered by something associated with it like a song, a smell or a place.

You also have certain thoughts that you think throughout the day, thoughts involving today's plans or a to-do list such as, *"I've got to get ready for that meeting. I have to pick up Emily at three. What should I fix for dinner"?*

Always beside or mixed in with these thoughts are some other thoughts that are with you throughout the day. These thoughts are always with you and are somewhat the same or similar and you think them every day. I like to call this your thought pattern, thought track and self-talk for it is a combination of all three.

Your thought pattern is the thoughts that make up the way you view yourself and the world around you and your relationship with it. That pattern has molded you into who and what you are. It is continually developing you into what you are becoming.

Your thought track is the way you talk to yourself and the general go to script you go by as you talk to yourself during the day, some would call it self-talk because it is the actual moment to moment conversation you are having with yourself throughout the day.

The pattern and track or self-talk is a reflection of what is going on within you. It reflects how you view yourself and where you place yourself in relation to everything else. How you view yourself in relation to the things going on around you and how they affect you. And the things you say in your head about the things that are actually happening to you or around you in the present. The thought pattern and the conversation you have with yourself goes on and is involved with the other tasks and activities you engage in as you go about your day. It all impacts you on multiple levels as every thought that you have has an impact upon you.

This pattern, track and the conversation you have with yourself changes and evolves ever so slowly. It has many different levels and layers. The tones, weight and shade of the thoughts and conversation within it changes depending on what you are going through and which direction you are moving in emotionally. But no matter what is going on it is almost the same day in and day out, and at the same time it is changing ever so slowly throughout your life because of the experiences you have and the choices you make.

Thoughts never stop, they are constant,
they are inescapable and because
of that they are the single most
overwhelming influence in our lives.

There are few of us that really choose what is on our thought track, for it develops or evolves as we live and experience life and all of the situations that come with daily activities. It changes constantly because it is affected by the things we are experiencing at any given moment in time and how we take that experience in. Then those experiences, and how we take them in, together with those things we hold onto and have allowed to develop into forces within us, are the factors that develop our patterns of thought, our thought track and our self-talk. All of those factors and forces that are a part of us continue to evolve and we evolve as we are influenced and created by them and with them, all of it happening and developing perpetually and unavoidably. It all happens, first in our immediate and daily living and then within and throughout our life.

Everything that you experience will have an effect on that thought pattern and thought track. The things said to you or done to you, and things you have done or said to others, how you are treated or were treated at times in your life. All of these things have had and will have an effect on that pattern and self-talk. They can have a profound and overwhelming influence upon you at the time that they happen and then can have a long term and healthy or unhealthy effect on you depending on how you take them in. It can also influence the way you view yourself in relation to everything else, because you won't or can't let it go.

If you are like most of us, because you are busy doing other things you don't really pay attention to what is going on in your mind. You spend most of the day on cruise control and just let your mind go. At certain times you become conscious of what is going on and what you are thinking, or you grab the controls and focus your conscious attention to be involved in a project, conversation or to problem solve. Sometimes you may catch yourself thinking something that you prefer not to think and say to yourself, "where did that come from", and try to let it go. These are conscious moments that we all have and we all have varying degrees of these moments and varying degrees of awareness of what we are thinking throughout the day.

It is the normal course of daily living that we kind of stay on cruise control and let that thought track roll.

Most of us are completely unaware of the power of the thoughts that are in our thought track. As our thoughts entertain us, they slowly designs and builds our life and our life experience. This all happens as we sit passive and unaware of the almost absolute power that our thoughts have in our lives, and we let them do it, unaware of what is really going on as they do so.

Most of us are almost completely unaware of the almost absolute power and influence that our thoughts have in our lives.

The life we have created by the thoughts that we think

Now consider your lifetime of experience and all of the things that you went through and how they each affected you. When you were a baby your mental slate was pure and clean. You accepted and trusted all that happened to you as a child because you knew full well that mother and father always had your best interests at heart. But as time went on things happened that may have started to bring that assumption into question.

As an example, maybe your little sister got the ice cream cone that you wanted and in your anger or because you weren't paying attention, you let the vanilla cone that you had been given began to drip all over the floor and the rug. Now you're catching hell and you have no reasonable understanding of how your mother could treat you like this.

Now your mind is starting to take on some color and depth. This experience that you just had is going be there in your mind to affect every perception and judgment and action, no matter how large or minute from that point on. Each and every thing said to you, everything done for you, against you or to you by everybody you interact with from this day forward is going to have to stand next to the ice cream incident and be subject to its influence as each of these experiences stand or shrink in its shadow. Then that experience, colored as it is by the ice cream incident, will take its place in your mind and be combined with the ice cream incident to color the next interaction, experience and any decision that happens in the endless interactions of daily life. And on and on and on and there is no way you or somebody else can ever get in your mind and fix it. You probably will never be able to remember it enough to pinpoint it as a cause anyway.

Our minds are filled up with these experiences, the good and pleasant, the bad and the ugly, meaningful and meaningless. All of them creating a kind of life mosaic that constantly regenerates and changes itself, forever changing and ever the same. Each of us is different because of many things, and one of the reasons we are different is because of these experiences and the way we string them together.

Every experience we have impacts our life and that impact is shaped, colored and has weight because of the way we hold onto it. This is the way it is, and we need to check our reality some of the time to make sure that an ice cream incident doesn't take over and dominate every experience and choice made from that day on.

Because it is impossible to think, talk or analyze our way out of the conditions these experiences have brought about, or to even identify them within ourselves, we can only know that negative forces and flaws are there within us along with all the good things.

Being still is a tool that helps to clear and purify the mind. It is a discipline that is effective in bringing things to the surface so that you can let them go, clearing your mind daily. It can be compared to the spiritual discipline of fasting in that as in fasting you deny the body the food it craves, in denying the body its normal food and water it allows it to rid itself of impurities and to give the digestive functions rest. So in being still you are denying the mind its appetite of holding onto and even hiding destructive thoughts and feelings.

As the thoughts in our mind entertain us,
they slowly design, create and build us
and our life, we let them do it, unaware
of what is really going on as they do so.

It gives the mind rest, it allows your conscious intelligent spirit a moment to step back from allowing the mind its tendency of building and reinforcing barriers to the self-realization of your potential. It is one of the advantages of the discipline and practice of Being Still that will enable you to recognize the barriers within you. As you calm your mind through the daily practice of Being Still it will clear and that will help you to see and identify these elements, then it is up to you to let them go.

Whether your life is a disaster or a beautiful experience you are forever affected by your history, your present thoughts and what you are expecting to happen in your future. Through the thoughts you allow into your mind you can have the power over what life will be like going forward. You now have the choice of changing your thoughts, what you think about and how you think. The control of almost your entire life presides in your thoughts. When you can learn to control your attention you can subdue your thoughts and have greater control of your life.

You cannot expect to change your life into a heavenly experience complete with fame and fortune and complete perfection because no matter how quickly and efficiently you change your thoughts you still have a history that influences you, complete with the karma you have created.

It is hard to change your thoughts when you do not know how the mind and thoughts work. If you are confused by the mental processes and it seems to be such a mystery, the prospect of changing your thoughts can be daunting. It can be fearsome when you are overwhelmed by them and wonder why the negative and destructive thoughts keep coming to mind even though you don't want them there.

Now that you understand some of the dynamics and the forces at play within your mind, you now have the power to change it. The mystery is gone, the power your mind has had over you, to overwhelm and control you, is shifted, that power is now in your hands because of the knowledge you have been given.

Do not let indecision, doubt or fear get in the way. Be confident in this knowledge and continue in your learning of how the mind really works.

Your mind and thoughts may work against you at this time because they want to maintain control, but I assure you that the realities that you are learning are true. But it is up to you to know for yourself that they are true or at least believe they are true for a time so that they become useful and powerful for you. If you have doubts you will need to test them out for yourself until you gain your own knowledge and understanding that they are true. Only by practicing the exercise of Being Still can you find out for yourself that they are true, I quote the Lord again, "be still and know", in order to know for yourself.

Thoughts really are the most powerful force in your life. Your attention is the food they need to sustain their life and existence, it is that simple. You will soon find that if you don't allow them your attention or a place in your mind they cannot survive as a controlling influence or force in your life.

Some of these concepts can seem as subtle as a thought itself, but reason will bear them out to be true.

Consciousness, mind and the mental process

How we are made

Now that you understand many of the dynamics and the things going on within the mind you have a better understanding of how the mind really works. And you know how depression, PTSD and things like panic attacks develop and happen. You know now that thoughts are the beginning, the foundation and the substance of everything.

The responsibility for your happiness or misery depends wholly upon the thoughts that you allow yourself to think and the thoughts that you allow to dominate your attention.

The science of this day would have us completely ignore the existence of the individual spirit within us. But we are more than mind and body, more than conscious and unconscious. We have to recognize the existence of our conscious and intelligent spirit to complete our knowledge and in order to gain a full understanding of ourselves and the whole mental process. Our conscious and intelligent spirit is at the center of who and what we are. We must know that it is the part and place within us that is the center of life, the light of our life, the purpose of our physical and mental existence and it encompasses our conscious existence. In order to fully understand ourselves and what is really going on within us we need to understand this.

These are key facts that have been continually overlooked or misunderstood by science, psychology, religion, and well, almost everybody. This knowledge will correct a basic flaw in our understanding of how we are designed, how we are made and how we, as human beings, function.

The critical fact that needs to be remembered is that that conscious intelligent part of us, our spirit, is not a part of or an extension of our mind, the mind is only a medium of experience and a tool of our conscious intelligent spirit. It is in fact like a lens that we experience life through.

The mental processes work differently than what is thought and taught. Many have assumed that thinking somehow just happens and we have no control over it or we have been given other explanations, such as it is the firing of synapses or electrical charges transferring between contact points in the brain. Another theory teaches that neuro-pathways are established that determines our actions and what is to be thought. None of these or any of the other theories regarding how the mind and thought works put forth so far by biology, psychology or any of the other sciences are reasonable. All are just theories and to continue in the established scientific lines of thinking there would exist no possibility of a cure for depression. Then a person's only hope to return to mental health would be to continue on this way and hope that time will heal.

We are less complicated, more importantly our mind and how it functions is less complicated than what we are taught to believe.

Have you ever asked yourself, what governs what is to be thought and how do we think a thought or what thought is to be thought? Do we leave that to a firing of a synapses or an electrical charge?

It is a certainty that if science continues to hold onto and cling to their lines of thinking they will never be able to define or answer basic questions about what really happens in the thinking processes.

Because science never recognizes the existence of the spirit and its essential place within us they will continue searching but will never be able to answer the questions, how are we made and how and what happens in the process of thinking a thought.

The brain is not the initiator or instigator of thoughts, except when related to bodily sensation such as vision, taste, noise, smell touch, pain or hunger.

Thinking happens differently than what science teaches and assumes. It has never been seriously considered how our mind and the thoughts within it really work. These questions have never been asked or addressed correctly. How do we think? What is going on in our heads when we think? How and what happens and why? What is the process of thinking a thought? And the universal question many of us asks, why am I having these thoughts that I don't want to think?

In order for thinking to happen there has to be an interaction or a communication between two things. That interaction happens between our conscious intelligent spirit and our mind. There has to be a presenter of the thought, which is what the mind does and a witness to the thought, which is what our conscious intelligent spirit does.

The thinking of a thought is an event or an interaction between these two separate parts of us, our mind and our conscious and intelligent spirit. Not unlike watching a movie we, our conscious spirit, is the viewer and the mind is the projecting equipment and the screen. The thoughts that the mind presents on the screen are like the scenes in the movie.

There has to exist a difference between you, the conscious

intelligent witness, and your mind for things to happen this way. Your intelligent spirit, your conscious witness, witnesses the event of the thought that is presented to you by your mind. When the mind presents the thought to your conscious spirit, your conscious spirit, the intelligent and conscious part of you, then processes the thought and the information the thought presents, Your conscious intelligent spirit, you, considers the information contained in the thought, combines it with any other information it has, makes a decision, then acts on it, stores it, waits for more information, or dismisses it. Your conscious spirit is the intelligent portion, the executive branch and the decision maker.

Mind is the recording and broadcasting, filming, filing and mechanical function of the mental processes. Mind has no innate intelligence beyond its capacity to present the thoughts to consciousness. That function is one of the natural processes of the mind, it is as much a natural process as the stomach digesting food. The mind is an inert substance dependent upon the light and life force of the conscious intelligent spirit.

The thinking process is the communication or interaction between your conscious intelligent spirit and your mind.

When you understand these concepts you soon realize that your mind is not god, nor is the mind all that you are, neither is the body who you are, you come in three parts, body, mind and spirit. Above all and foremost you are a spirit, a conscious intelligent spiritual being that uses your body and your mind to gain knowledge, experience and to interact and function in life.

For many of us the mind seems to be such a mystery. Because it appears to be so vast and to have so much power we are daunted by it. Almost like the ocean or outer space, we are in awe of what may be out there and within its vastness. But the apparent vastness and mysteries of the mind are only because of our lack of understanding and the perception we hold. In fact the mind is not the powerful, vast and infinite thing within you, it is merely a medium of experience, it is the lens that you experience life through. It is your spirit that is the powerful, vast, infinite and immortal part of you. It is your spirit and not your mind that has vast, unlimited and infinite capacity and potential.

In fact, the expression and realization of all of the power and capacity of your spirit is hindered or limited by what your thoughts and mind convinces you that your limits are. Your shortcomings are shortcomings of the mind and not you or the conscious and intelligent spirit that you are. Your confusion and inability to cope is because of the confusion that is in your mind.

The mind is the lens that your spirit experiences life through and like any lens, if it is colored or blurred or if it is out of focus, it will distort everything you see and experience and with these conditions your perceptions and understanding of things can be untrue or at least skewed.

All of these shortcomings, confusion and seeming lack of power to control what is happening to you is because you have misunderstood and have let your mind become supreme ruler over you. Your mind rules over you and has its way because you are convinced that there is nothing that you can do to correct it, you allow this because you have believed it is all powerful. But the reality is that the mind will only have as much power as you allow it to have once you understand what it is and how it really interacts with your spirit. You need to understand the minds place and its function within you. Then you must learn and practice a little self-discipline in order to take back control of it.

Thoughts are the most influential
and powerful force in all of
creation and within our life.

Realities of Mental Dynamics

Our life is created, formed and governed by the continued and unending thinking of our thoughts. The time that is not spent consciously thinking about something or engaged in a conversation or concentrating on a project is filled up with other, idle thoughts that can be constructive, unconstructive or even destructive to our being.

A large factor in this type of other thoughts that we think is influenced by what we are going through and the direction we are moving in emotionally. Many people control their other thoughts because they are engaged in a reasonably good life with job and family. Because they are somewhat engaged in the business of living that life, it keeps them emotionally stable and secure and the thoughts they entertain are somewhat true and constructive. At the very least the constructive and positive thoughts outweigh the negative and destructive thoughts that are moving through their mind.

But things can happen to us, or can happen in our life, that can turn our thinking or change the ratios of positive and negative thoughts. Life events such as, emotional trauma, feeling overwhelmed or having some kind of loss or other sudden life changes will alter our thinking and emotional condition for a time. The things and events that can cause this are too numerous to mention. Things such as loss of someone close to us, a divorce, loss of a job, almost anything that causes an emotional turmoil in life. The point is that life happens and the experiences we have in life and the things we go through makes changes in us and the way we think and all of those things will affect us mentally and emotionally.

Most times we will recover naturally from difficult life experiences and changes in a relatively short time. The emotional turmoil the experience causes will pass and we then return to normal, our confidence and positive self-image remains intact. As we deal with the difficulty in a positive manner we receive the benefit of deeper spiritual understanding because every experience we have brings about a more understanding of ourselves and life.

Hard times in life are sometimes for that purpose, to bring about growth in us from the lessons that they teach. Some would even say that, we should rejoice in the face of calamity because it means that something is happening in our life. The more difficult the situation and experience, the more growth we have and the deeper our understanding of life is. It is the experiences in life that is the reason we are here, what we learn from them is what gives us spiritual growth and wisdom. Some say that even the bad things we endure, when viewed from an eternal perspective are for our spiritual benefit.

However, sometimes these experiences seem to be too much for us to handle and we don't recover the way we should. We allow our thinking, our thought pattern and our self-talk to go negative and they remain negative long enough that we find that we reach

Lies and fantasies have no foundation in reality, they are like smoke, as we continuously remove our attention from them they will dissipate into nothing.

a point where we cannot reverse the trend in the natural course of life and living. No amount thinking, talking or therapy is bringing us back to our old self with our own confidence and positive outlook on life. We have come to a point where we have lost control of our thoughts. The thoughts we now have and our emotions have taken over and overwhelmed us. We are now in a place where our thoughts rule and they have deteriorated into a self-destructive mental funk and along with those overwhelming and intrusive thoughts we are having, we find ourselves on an emotional roller coaster.

This is the point where the mind, yes the mind and the negative and untrue thoughts about ourselves have literally taken over our life. Our thoughts are in a downward spiral from which we can no longer regain control. These negative and self-destructive thoughts we are having, have now become stronger and more permanent within the thought patterns that we spend our day in. We have become depressed.

Almost like a movie reel or an audio tape, the same thoughts and patterns of thoughts that have developed keep coming into our mind. Those thoughts and thought patterns become so embedded in our mind that they are the only things that we think about all day and night. We are unavoidably feeding them as they constantly intrude themselves into our mental processes. From the morning when we awake we find ourselves in perpetual negative self-analysis and negative self-discussion and we cannot seem to change it.

Now, the thought pattern that keeps rolling through our mind is almost always the same day after day. It has become like a reel of tape showing the same movie with a voice print of negative self-discussion that we cannot seem to change, and it will not stop.

Thoughts are created things and they exist within the mind, and their existence does not depend on or matter whether the thought is true or not. Thoughts that are not true are destructive and given enough time and attention will affect our perception of reality and even become our reality. Remember this; it is the thoughts which contain the lies that are the ones that are most aggressive in seeking our attention. The thoughts that we give our attention to become strong and powerful over time and they will not go away.

What develops from this condition is almost like a thought forest that we have allowed to be created and has grown up around us. The thoughts that now make up our present pattern of thought are wild, uncontrolled and perpetual and we are lost in them. We are not going to think our way out of the forest; we are not going to talk our way out of it either. In fact, remember that the more we think or talk about them, the more power we give them and as we think the thoughts and try to solve the problem in this way the denser the forest becomes and the more confused and lost we become.

The only complete and permanent way out is by cutting down the forest, destroying the thoughts and freeing ourselves through our own efforts. That takes knowledge and understanding of the mind and of how to control our attention. We now know that by just controlling our attention and refusing to think those thoughts we have the power to destroy the negative thinking pattern we have become lost and ensnared in.

When your thoughts are on the business of living, instead of constant negative self-analysis, then you know you have your life back.

THE EFFECTS OF
YOUR ATTENTION

**Remember,
even those intrusive thoughts can
only exist because you think them.**

Truth and Lies

We have two primary types or classes of thoughts that exist in our mind, those two classes are truth and lies.

Thoughts that are true and that are based on reality such as facts, experience and acquired knowledge exist on their own, they have their own foundation therefore they do not need our attention to exist. Truth and reality exists independent of our attention and our conception. Therefore thoughts and impressions that are true and real do not need, nor do they seek our attention.

Lies are a type of thoughts that exists only because we think them.

When we think thoughts about ourselves that are not true, thoughts that cause doubt and anxiety in us are usually lies. When we give thoughts such as these any degree of our attention, we are giving them life. When we think these thoughts we are feeding them with mental energy, or the energy of mind. When we think them, our attention directs mental energy into them, which sustains and feeds them. These types of thoughts need our mental energy to exist and they cannot exist without it.

Untrue thoughts will begin their existence by coming to mind when we are not really paying attention to what we are thinking about at the time. Before we became depressed, the self-defeating and self-effacing and debasing type thoughts didn't really bother us in the way they do now. We had confidence in ourselves and who we were, and we were able to dismiss negative thoughts about ourselves out of hand. We knew they were untrue and refused to give them a second moment of our attention. In the process of becoming depressed we allowed them some of our attention, maybe we gave them a second of consideration. Then we gave them more and more of our attention. At some point in our descent into depression, not only did we allow ourselves to think them more, but we even began to examine them and wondered if they were true, or we have come to even believe that they are true.

These are lies about ourselves that we allow ourselves to think. We all have them, fears about the way we look, what people are thinking and saying about us or to us. Then even more damaging are the negative comments we say to ourselves about ourselves, such as, "I'm not good enough, I'm a stupid, ugly, loser".

Before we got depressed we dismissed these lies about ourselves and they remained weak and ineffectual because of it. As we started to get down and bummed out and as depression started to set in, we may still have been able to dismiss them. But to some degree we wondered, now and then, if they were true. Because of that little attention and wondering, we were giving them some strength and with that strength, they were able to come back around and to get some more of our attention.

"We sit by and let our thoughts entertain us, unaware that those thoughts and the words and the concepts we think are in fact creating our whole life and the life we experience."

Even though we will dismiss these thoughts again and again, at the moment we are a bit down, we give them a little bit more of our attention and when we do that they are fed and strengthened just a little or to the degree of attention we gave to them. Then that thought will come around more because it has received a little attention and with it substance and strength from the mental energy we fed into it.

By continuing this activity, over time they can and will eventually gain enough strength and power to come back around more often. As we allow and even cause that to happen it gains enough of a foothold that it becomes embedded in our mind, even as we are questioning in our mind if the lie is true, it is absorbing energy. Then as the thought grows in substance from our attention, we may even begin to believe that it is true. As that happens it continues to grow stronger and more powerful and comes around so much that eventually we cannot control or dismiss it anymore. Then comes the tipping point in this process where the thoughts become uncontrollable and intrusive.

The only reason that the thoughts exist, the only reason they have substance and power is because of our attention, because we think them.

Isn't it interesting that even on a good day it is often the negative, self-diminishing thoughts about yourself that seem to surface and come into your mind and causes you to doubt. Have you ever asked yourself, why that is?

The Effects of your Attention

To give you a practical example of how lies can gain a place in your mind and become intrusive is best demonstrated by something that we have all done, fantasized.

All of us have fanaticized at one time or another. We have fanaticized about saving the day, being a hero, winning a contest or a sporting event. We have also had romantic or sexual fantasies at one time or another.

Fantasies are all fundamentally the same in that they are all just thoughts. All of our fantasies differ in subject matter and content but their common denominator is that they are all made of thoughts that are untrue. Fantasies are thoughts that have no foundation in truth. Because they have no foundation in truth or reality their existence is dependent upon our thinking them and the attention we give to them as we are thinking them. Unless or until we give our fantasy some sustaining attention they remain just fleeting thoughts and they just disappear into nothingness.

But we sometimes have that certain fantasy that we enjoy thinking about and spending some time with.

Now in creating your fantasy remember how you spent some time conjuring it up and then spent time entertaining yourself with it, revisiting it over the course of a few days or longer.

Thoughts become intrusive in the same way a fantasy that you have thought about too much does. You've thought about it so much that when you decided not to think about it anymore it just doesn't immediately go away. Remember how you had to consciously avoid thinking about it for a few days for it to stop coming back?

Then after a while, realizing what a waste of time it was, you decided to stop thinking about it. Did it instantly disappear from your mind? No, in most instances it did not. In fact, you had to put forth some effort in trying to avoid thinking the fantasy or the thoughts of the fantasy. Over time, perhaps a few days, you avoided the thoughts and the fantasy slowly lost the power to come back.

Now the reason that it kept coming into your mind is because it had gathered enough substance and power from your attention that it could not easily be dismissed. It wouldn't just go away because it had gained enough substance and strength from your attention and effectively became embedded in your mind. Then, having become a thing of substance, it continued to seek your attention to maintain its existence.

How Depression Takes Hold

What happened with the fantasy is the same thing that happens with all thoughts that you think multiple times or thoughts that you continue to dwell on. The attention that you gave to it when thinking about it, the stronger and more established and imbedded in your mind it became. Because of the strength and power that your attention allowed the thoughts to absorb and build, the more time it took to dissolve or to shrink the power it had to come back to or to stay in your mind. This is a dynamic of mind, this is the way thoughts and thinking works and this is an aspect of the way the entire mind and thought processes work.

That may sound too simple but it really is that simple. This should help you to understand how mind, thoughts and thinking works, how intrusive thoughts became intrusive and how you can became overwhelmed and depressed because of them.

The more attention you give a thought and the more frequent you think it, the stronger and more imbedded in your mind it becomes. This explains and demonstrates to us, how fantasies can become so embedded in the mind that they become hard to get rid of. This also demonstrates how the lies and negative self-effacing type thinking and thoughts, the kind that cause depression, become embedded in your mind and how those thoughts increasingly grow strong and intrusive because you have continued to think them and talk about them.

Intrusiveness of thought develops in the same way as fantasies develop, given enough attention there comes a point where you can't stop thinking them. They develop by accumulating the mental energies you direct into them as you think them. They seek and gather the substance and power to stay in your mind from the mental energy your attention directs into them. It happens in the same way as a fantasy, only because you think them.

Because lies have no foundation
in truth or reality they need your
attention to exist, and it should not be
a mystery why it is those thoughts that
continually come into your mind.

Like everything else thoughts are a part of creation and like every other thing in creation thoughts are either generating or degenerating. Any thoughts that we give our attention to will generate, it will grow and strengthen in correlation to the degree of attention we give to them. Very simply, the more we think them, the stronger they get. Conversely, the moment we begin to deny them our attention they begin to degenerate and their power to come back is diminished.

Through this example we have established that it is the lies and fantasy type thoughts that are the greatest cause of depression, they are the self-defeating and negative forces that dwell in the mind. They are the thoughts that will continually try to come into your mind seeking your attention because that gives them sustenance, which provides for their existence and eventual power. As you give them your attention they will grow and become stronger and more intrusive.

Because lies and fantasy thoughts are the type of thoughts that have no foundation in truth or reality they need your attention to exist, and it should not be a mystery that it is those thoughts that continually try to come into your mind. You know that they do that in order to exist and sustain themselves. If they are successful at continually coming into your mind, these lies and fantasies can and will become so powerful that they can even redefine the reality that you perceive.

How Lies and Fantasy Can Become Our Reality

Because of this dynamic, there are people that can become so departed from what is real that the substance of their life experience has less and less to do with reality.

Jill is a prime example, she is 14 years old and one day as she was walking down the hall of her school she heard a whisper, spoken by one of the other girls in the school hallway just loud enough for Jill to hear. The whisperer says, "look at how fat Jill is getting".

Because of the way people sometimes are and the motivations they have we can all relate to a scene like that. We have all heard of or seen similar things happen, maybe even to us.

The truth is that Jill is not fat and she knows it, she is in fact blossoming into a beautiful young woman. But later that day Jill checks herself in the mirror. Seeing that she isn't fat she dismisses the thought and the whisper she heard. But over the next few days she finds herself hearing that whisper in her head. Because of it she keeps checking her weight. The very thought of her being fat is a thought that she finds herself thinking again and again, constantly entertaining.

Sometimes reason and intelligence is not enough to overcome what we know in our mind and heart is a lie.

Soon she is hyperaware of what she eats. Very soon she is skipping breakfast and lunch and pushing the food around her plate at dinner to hide the fact that she isn't eating. Now weeks later she has lost a lot of weight, but even now, as she is wasting away because of lack of nourishment, she is looking in the mirror constantly and when she does, she is only seeing how fat she is. Eventually she is down to 50 LBS or less, she is skin and bones, but she has convinced herself that she is fat.

How can she be skin and bones and stand in front of a mirror and see herself as grossly overweight? It is because she has given so much attention to the untrue thoughts about herself that they have literary become her reality. Although false, the thoughts or image of herself being fat have become so real to her that they have become a part of the substance or reality of her life and experience. Remember the lens that you experience life through?

This is an extreme but true example, one of many instances we have all heard about that demonstrates how lies and fantasy and false thoughts can become powerfully real in the mind. It demonstrates the power of thoughts and how they can become an overwhelming influence in a life, even when not true. Jill is not alone, because we all have some degree of false realities in our mind.

In much the same way that Jill has been subdued and convinced by a false reality, we can also become subject to an experience that seems to be real but is not. For example how unreasonable are the thoughts that a person has during a panic attack. They are just thoughts and we know it even as it is happening, but we are so carried away with fear that these thoughts and emotions bring with them that we cannot control what is happening. In this and other ways our experience can parallel what Jill is going through.

In the beginning of Jill's departure from reality, she knew that what was said was not true. But the whisperer's words became embedded in her mind and thought process, becoming intrusive as she started to believe that they were true.

Sometimes reason and intelligence is not enough to overcome

what we know intellectually and reasonably is a lie. In some instances we cannot think or reason our way out, in fact that just exacerbates the problem. In situations like these, in order to free ourselves, we have to let go of the thoughts themselves, we have to force ourselves to stop thinking them.

When we make the effort and use some mental discipline when dealing with all of these, the lies, the fear, the doubt, the emotions and the flood of fear that comes with a panic attack, we find that by just holding the mind still and breathing will help us to get past it and diminish its effects. Over time and consistent daily practice of the Being Still discipline, these types of problems will disappear altogether. The more we use this method the more effective it becomes in freeing ourselves from these types of problems.

"The light of a candle does not
flicker in a windless place"

Bhagavad Gita

Overcoming fear, doubt and emotions

Refusing to think the thought and holding the mind still does much more than just take away the power of the thought to exist. As the thoughts lose their power to return, they are no longer able to bring the forces that accompany them. Forces such as fear, doubt, emotions, panic and any other feeling or experience that accompanies the thought is denied also.

Any of the circumstances or experience the thoughts have helped create will lose the power and influence over us because they need our attention to the thought it accompanies. It is the thought that brings the fear and the emotion along with it. In all cases the existence and power of a feeling such as fear is wholly dependent on the thought or the thoughts the fear and emotion accompanies.

Let us reason together
for a moment;

Now let's approach this from another way. You have been continually thinking the thoughts that your mind keeps presenting to you, mostly because you didn't think you had a choice. Up to this point your mind has completely ruled over you in this way. Now I want you to consider what would happen if you could ignore the thoughts your mind presented to you to think. Consider what would happen if you could deny those thoughts a place in your mind and just let go of them? What will happen if every time you had a thought try to enter your mind you let it go and refused to think it or dwell on it, especially thoughts that are untrue and self-effacing or the kind of thoughts that cause negative emotions and such things as fear or anger? As impossible as it may seem at this point, can you imagine the result of doing that for any length of time, if you were able? Wouldn't it bring about a completely calm, clear and unfettered mind, a mind void of the emotional turmoil, depressive thoughts and the emotions they bring with them? If you could do that, if you could stop thinking those thoughts, nothing could bother you because nothing would interrupt your peace or bring fear or negative emotion into your experience.

In the Sanskrit there is a passage that says, **"The light of a candle does not flicker in a windless place". In this passage, the light of the candle represents your conscious intelligent spirit and that windless place is a calm, clear and peaceful mind.**

This is a picture or illustration of a perfect mental place. It probably describes what most people would think of having "peace of mind". A place where the cares and disappointments in life and daily living will not bother us because of a calm and peaceful mind. A calm and peaceful mind is also a clear mind, able to see and know things as they really are.

"By small and simple means are great things brought to pass: and small means in many instances doth confound the wise."

Alma,
A Book of Mormon Prophet

Knowledge is Power

Until we understand our condition we will never be free of it. In our ignorance we will continue to constantly think and talk about the thoughts, not realizing that the very talking, thinking and the self-analysis that we spend our whole day in is, in fact, feeding and strengthening the uncontrolled and intrusive type thoughts that contribute to our problem.

Before now you really didn't know what was really going on in your mind and that what you were likely doing to overcome the problem was working against you and just made the problem worse.

Without Being Still your condition will self-perpetuate and then, if possible, only time can heal. And even then, without this knowledge of what is really going on, even as you get better you would be forever threatened, worrying that you could slip back into depression.

You need to realize that you can't have it both ways, that you can't spend all of your time thinking and talking about something and then expect it to suddenly go away or even to go away at all. Along with the strengthening of the intrusive thoughts, all of that thinking and talking about it increases your confusion and draws you deeper into depression. Everything you are doing is contributing to the downward spiral as you struggle to try and figure yourself out.

The more you talk and think about it, searching for these imagined triggers or unresolved issues you will just go deeper into the woods of confusion. Even if you could somehow figure it all out, if there really was a deep psychological problem and you could pinpoint and identify it, then what, is there a pill? And even if there was a pill for that, then what? You still wouldn't be healed and neither would your condition be substantially improved because of the energy of mind your attention has fed into the confusion of your thoughts. And the thoughts and the confusion will not just go away without having an effective method of removing them.

The mystery is gone, the power your mind has had over you, to overwhelm and control you, is shifted, that power is now yours because of the knowledge you now have. Be confident in that knowledge. Do not let indecision, doubt or fear get in the way. The knowledge you have is real, reason proves it. Some time spent Being Still will provide you with further proof and you will feel much better.

To the mind that is still...

The whole universe surrenders

Lao Tzu

About the Author

Doug Zaccanelli is married; he and his wife Carol have three grown children together. They live in an old farmhouse beside a lake in Michigan.

Doug has been practicing and teaching a discipline called Raja Yoga since the early 1970's. He came upon it while searching for a way out of the deep depression and post traumatic stress he was in after his time as a combat infantryman in Vietnam.

Raja Yoga involves training the mind, using progressive and sometimes intense breathing exercises together with concentration techniques that are designed to help calm and still the mind. From the mental training and the intense discipline, Raja Yoga also becomes a study of consciousness, mind and thoughts and their processes. In the course of his studies he discovered some simple realities of mind and thought that are not obvious and many have overlooked.

The most important discovery he has found is that there is healing power in holding the mental processes still. Holding the mind and mental processes still and stopping thought is the purpose of practicing Raja Yoga. The activity of stopping thoughts and the thought processes affects the thoughts that cause depression. The process quickly and effectively breaks down the intrusive and overwhelming thoughts and thought patterns that depressed people find themselves in.

Being still is based on the broader discipline of Raja Yoga, but with the central focus on a simple mental exercise of holding the mental processes still. While teaching Being Still he has continued to perfect the exercise. In the end, what he teaches has become a very short and simple mental exercise. This system is so simple that it will enable almost anyone to use it successfully. It has been proven successful for everyone who practices it.

Since 2008 Mr. Zaccanelli has been teaching his Being Still exercise to military veterans at the Battle Creek Veterans Hospital. Some of what is covered in this book is based on the things he teaches at the VA Hospital.

Mr. Zaccanelli has spent many years counseling, teaching and researching the causes and cures for depression and PTSD. As he explains in this work, depression and PTSD is because of the conscious thoughts and not some subconscious or unconscious thing, as many believe. His extensive research and personal experience makes him able to explain how and why that is. He is able to explain what is really going on in the mind and how it works. His knowledge and experience make him uniquely qualified and able to teach these correct principles in a way that most people can understand and will make them better able to free themselves from their condition.

dougzaccanelli@gmail.com
www.stopthethoughts.org